C000212277

KETOGENIC

DIET

Ketogenic Diet: A Beginner's Guide to Lose Fat
and Get Healthy With High-fat Foods

**A Fast and Simple Guide to Lose Weight and Live
Healthier**

@ Timmy Bell

Published By Adam Gilbin

@ Timmy Bell

Ketogenic Diet: A Beginner's Guide to Lose Fat
and Get Healthy With High-fat Foods

**A Fast and Simple Guide to Lose Weight and Live
Healthier**

ISBN 978-1-990053-27-6

TABLE OF CONTENTS

Delightful Scrambled Eggs

Ingredients:

- Coarse Salt

- Fresh Ground Pepper

- 3 Large Eggs

- 1 tablespoon of Unsalted Butter

Directions:

1. Beat your eggs using your fork.
2. Melt your butter using a nonstick medium skillet over a low heat.
3. Add in your egg mixture.
4. Using your spatula (preferably flexible and heatproof), gently move your eggs into the

center of your pan and allow the liquid parts
to run out to the perimeter.

5. Continue to cook moving your eggs with your
    spatula until they are set.

6. Should take approximately 1 1/2 minutes to 3
    minutes.

7. Season your eggs with your pepper and salt.

8. Serve!

Keto Bacon Pancakes

Ingredients:

- 1 tablespoon of Sugar-Free Vanilla Syrup

- 1/2 cup of Melted Unsalted Butter

- 1 cup of Carbquik

- 1/2 teaspoon of Baking Soda

- 1 Egg

- 1/2 cup of Heavy Cream

- 8 slices of Bacon

- 1/4 cup of Water

Directions:

1. Cook your bacon.

2. Melt your butter in your microwave.

3. Mix together your baking soda and Carbquik.

4. Add your liquid ingredients and mix it all
    together.

5. Heat your pan over a medium-high heat.
    Spray it with Pam.

6. Spoon some batter into your pan. Don't make
    the pancake so large you can't flip it. Add your
    bacon.

7. When your edges brown or bubbles form in
    the center flip your pancake.

8. Continue to cook for another minute until the
    center is cooked.

9. Check with your fork.

10. Remove your pancakes and make the next
    one.

11. Repeat the process until all your pancakes are
    finished.

12. Serve!

Raspberry Protein Pancakes

Ingredients:

- 2 tablespoons of Almond Milk

- 2 tablespoons of Greek Yogurt

- 3/4 cup of Raspberries

- 1 tablespoon of Chia Seeds

- 1/4 cup of Egg Whites

- 1 scoop of Whey Protein Powder

- 1/2 Banana

- 1 tablespoon of Cinnamon

Directions:

1. Mash up your banana.

2. Grind up your chia seeds.

3. Add all your ingredients except your raspberries to your bowl and stir together well.

4. Add your raspberries and stir.

5. Spray your small-sized pan with some olive oil spray and then pour in your mix.

6. Cook your pancakes on a medium heat until your edges are brown. Once this occurs flip your pancakes.

7. Continue cooking until the middle has been well cooked. Check with your fork.

8. Add to your plate along with your Greek yogurt.

9. Serve!

Pumpkin Cream Cheese Pancakes

Ingredients:

Pancakes:

- 2 ounces of Cream Cheese

- 1/4 tablespoon of Pumpkin Pie Spice

- 2 Eggs

- 2 tablespoons of Coconut Flour

Pumpkin Butter:

- 1/2 tablespoon of 100% Pumpkin

- 3 tablespoons of Unsalted Butter

- 1/16 teaspoon of Raw Stevia

Directions:

1. Mix together your pumpkin and butter. Microwave for intervals of 10 seconds until it is smooth.
2. Once it's smooth, add in your Stevia for taste.
3. Next work on pancakes.
4. Mix your eggs, cream cheese, pumpkin pie spice, and coconut flour until blended together.
5. Heat your non-stick pan over a medium heat. Add a tablespoon of butter.
6. When your butter begins to brown add in half of your pancake mix.
7. Once your edges brown or the center bubbles, flip your pancake.
8. Cook for around 1 minute or until the center is cooked.
9. Check with your fork.

10. Remove from your pan and add to your plate.

11. Repeat this process with your next pancake.

12. Once all your pancakes are done add your pumpkin butter.

13. Serve!

Squash Spaghetti Pancakes

Ingredients:

- 1 teaspoon of Onion Powder

- 1 teaspoon of Garlic Powder

- 1 teaspoon of Salt

- 1 teaspoon of Pepper

- 10 ounces of Cooked Spaghetti Squash

- 2 Eggs

- 1 ounce of Parmesan Cheese

- 4 slices of Thick Cut Bacon

Directions:

1. Cook your spaghetti squash.

10

2. Cook your bacon until it's crispy.

3. Add your eggs, spices, cheese, and spaghetti squash to your bowl and mix.

4. Crumble your bacon and add it to your mixture.

5. Heat your bacon grease in the skillet until they are shimmering.

6. Scoop your mixture into bacon grease. Make four piles and then use a spatula to compress your piles flat.

7. After bottom begins to brown flip it.

8. You can add a dollop of sour cream or some chives if you want.

9. Serve!

Keto French Toast

Ingredients:

- 1/4 cup of Fresh Whole Butter

- 1 tablespoon of Swerve or Sugar Equivalent

- 1/2 cup of Heavy Whipping Cream

- Pinch of Salt

- 8 Large Eggs

- 3/4 cup of Unsweetened Almond Milk

- 2 teaspoon of Baking Powder

- 1/4 cup of Coconut Flour

- 1 teaspoon of Vanilla Extract

- 1/4 cup of Melted Butter

Directions:

1. Mix your coconut flour, baking powder, salt, and sugar.
2. In a different bowl, whisk together 4 of your 8 eggs. Add 1/4 cup of your almond milk and vanilla. Whisk together.
3. Add your dry and wet ingredients together and whisk. Continue to do so while pouring in your melted butter.
4. Grease your 12 microwave safe containers. Use wide containers.
5. Microwave your muffins. For each additional muffin add a minute to your microwave time. I made 2 batches of 6 muffins with 6 minutes for each batch.
6. While your muffins are cooking, in your large-sized mixing bowl, whisk together your other

4 eggs, 1/2 cup of heavy cream, and 1/2 cup of almond milk.

7. As muffins come out of your microwave, pop them out of containers and allow them to cool for a minute.

8. When they are cool enough, add to your egg mixture and allow them to sit for a couple minutes.

9. Flip them occasionally while letting them sit.

10. Once they've absorbed some of your mixture, heat up your large-sized skillet over a medium-low heat. Add some fresh butter and melt it.

11. Fry your muffins like you would French toast.

12. Serve!

Goulash soup

Ingredients:

- 100 ml white wine, dry

- 400 ml beef broth

- salt

- pepper

- Paprika powder

- chili

- 1 teaspoon mustard

- 1 pickle, chopped, without sugar

- 1 clove of garlic, chopped

- 250 g beef goulash

- 2 onions, cut into quarters

- 1 red pepper, diced

- 1 yellow pepper, diced

- 200 g mushrooms, cut into quarters

- 50 g tomato paste

Directions:

1. Heat a saucepan and add the meat with the mustard, the pickled cucumber and the onions, peppers, mushrooms and the garlic to fry.

2. Add the beef broth, white wine, tomato paste, and spices and stir well.

3. Now let the goulash simmer for 60 minutes over a low heat.

Pizza pan with bacon

Ingredients:

- 100 g rocket

- 4 tbsp tomatoes, happened

- 1 onion, cut into rings

- 8 slices of bacon

- pepper

- 2 teaspoons of oregano

- salt

- 4 tbsp water

- 80 g coconut flour

- 4 egg whites

- 2 eggs

- 1 green pepper, cut into strips

- 100 g cheese, grated

Directions:

1. Mix the egg whites, two eggs, coconut flour, water, pepper, salt and oregano.
2. Take the dough and press it into the pan, put the lid on.
3. Let the dough bake for 4 minutes, turn it over and bake it again for 2 minutes.
4. Brush the dough with the tomatoes.
5. Cover the dough with the ingredients, except for the rocket.
6. Close the lid again and cook for another 3 minutes.
7. Then sprinkle everything with the rocket and serve.

Mince pan

Ingredients:

- oregano

- nutmeg

- Paprika powder

- Garlic powder

- 2 onions, chopped

- 300 g parsley root

- 250 g ground beef

- salt

- pepper

Directions:

1. Heat a pan and add the minced meat with the spices and onion.

2. Fry everything.

3. Take the parsley root and peel it, then cut it into slices.

4. Take minced meat out of the pan.

5. Put the slices of parsley root in the pan and let them fry for 15 minutes.

6. Add the minced meat again, heat briefly and serve.

Chicory casserole

Ingredients:

- 100 ml soy cream

- 1 teaspoon oil

- salt

- pepper

- nutmeg

- Paprika powder

- 2 tbsp oregano

- Chilli flakes

- 3 eggs

- 200 g turkey breast fillet, cut into cubes

- 1 onion, chopped

- 100 g mushrooms, quartered

- 300 g chicory

- 20 g parmesan, grated

- 1 clove of garlic, pressed

- 100 ml coconut milk

Directions:

1. Clean the chicory and cut it into individual leaves.
2. Switch the oven to 180 ° C fan oven and prepare a baking dish.
3. Heat the oil in a pan and fry the meat with the spices in it.
4. Add the vegetables.

5. Mix the eggs, milk and cream, season everything and let it steep for a moment.
6. Put the chicory in the baking dish and cover it with the contents of the pan.
7. Scatter the parmesan on top and let the casserole bake for 30 minutes.

Cauliflower casserole

Ingredients:

- 2 tbsp flaxseed flour

- 2 tbsp coconut flour

- 2 tbsp butter, for frying

- 2 tbsp butter, melted

- salt

- pepper

- nutmeg

- 300 ml coconut milk, from a can

- 400 g cauliflower, frozen

- 200 g minced meat

- 150 g Emmentaler cheese, grated

- 1 onion, chopped

- 12 g ginger, grated

- 2 cloves of garlic, chopped

Directions:

1. Take a large saucepan of salted water and pre-cook the cauliflower for 3 minutes.
2. Switch the oven to 180 ° C fan oven. Prepare a baking dish.
3. Put the minced meat with the butter, onions and garlic and ginger in a pan, fry together with the spices.
4. Stir in the coconut flour and let it thicken briefly.
5. Extinguish with the coconut milk and take the pot off the stove.

6. Fill the cauliflower into the pan and cover it with the contents of the pan.

7. Mix the flaxseed, parmesan and 2 tablespoons of melted butter well, then pour the mixture over the casserole.

8. Cook this in the oven for 25-30 minutes.

Chicken Parmigiana

Ingredients:

- Salt and ground black pepper, as required

- 4 -6-ounces grass-fed skinless, boneless chicken breasts, pounded into a ½-inch thickness

- ¼ cup olive oil

- 1½ cups marinara sauce

- 4 ounces mozzarella cheese, thinly sliced

- 2 tablespoons fresh parsley, chopped

- 1 large organic egg, beaten

- ½ cup of superfine blanched almond flour

- ¼ cup Parmesan cheese, grated

- ½ teaspoon dried parsley

- ½ teaspoon paprika

- ½ teaspoon garlic powder

Directions:

1. Preheat the oven to 375 degrees F.
2. Add the beaten egg into a shallow dish.
3. Place the almond flour, Parmesan, parsley, spices, salt, and black pepper in another shallow dish and mix well.
4. Dip each chicken breast into the beaten egg and then coat with the flour mixture.
5. Heat the oil in a deep skillet over medium-high heat and fry the chicken breasts for about 3 minutes per side.

6. Using a slotted spoon, moved the chicken breasts onto a paper towel-lined plate to drain.

7. At the bottom of a casserole, put about ½ cup of marinara sauce and spread evenly.

8. Arrange the chicken breasts over marinara sauce in a single layer.

9. Top with the remaining marinara sauce, followed by mozzarella cheese slices.

10. Bake for about at least 20 minutes or until done completely.

11. Take off from the oven and serve hot with the garnishing of fresh parsley.

Shrimp Risotto

Ingredients:

- ½ lemon

- 4 stalks green onion

- 3 tbsp. ghee butter

- 2 tbsp. coconut oil

- Salt and black pepper to taste

- 14 oz. shrimps, peeled and deveined

- 12 oz. cauli rice

- 4 button mushrooms

Directions:

1. Preheat the oven to 400F

2. Put a layer of cauli rice on a sheet pan, season with salt and spices; sprinkle the coconut oil over it
3. Bake in the oven for 10-12 minutes
4. Cut the green onion, slice up the mushrooms and remove the rind from the lemon
5. Heat the ghee butter in a skillet over medium heat. Add the shrimps; season it and sauté for 5-6 minutes
6. Top the cauli rice with the shrimps, sprinkle the green onion over it

Lemony Trout

Ingredients:

- 1 tsp rosemary

- 1 lemon

- 2 tbsp. capers

- Salt and pepper to taste

- 5 tbsp. ghee butter

- 5 oz. trout fillets

- 2 garlic cloves

Directions:

1. Preheat the oven to 400F

2. Peel the lemon, mince the garlic cloves and chop the capers

3. Season the trout fillets with salt, rosemary, and pepper

4. Grease a baking dish with the oil and place the fish onto it

5. Warm the butter in a skillet over medium heat

6. Add the garlic and cook for 4-5 minutes until golden

7. Remove from the heat, add the lemon zest and 2 tablespoons of lemon juice, stir well

8. Pour the lemon-butter sauce over the fish and top with the capers

9. Bake for 14-15 minutes. Serve hot

Quick Fish Bowl

Ingredients:

- 1 tbsp. ghee butter

- 1 tbsp. cumin powder

- 1 tbsp. paprika

- 2 cups coleslaw cabbage, chopped

- 1 tbsp. salsa sauce

- Himalayan rock salt, to taste

- Black pepper to taste

- 2 tilapia fillets

- 1 tbsp. olive oil

- 1 avocado

Directions:

1. Preheat the oven to 425F. Line a baking sheet with the foil
2. Mash the avocado
3. Brush the tilapia fillets using olive oil, season with salt and spices
4. Place the fish onto the baking sheet, greased with the ghee butter
5. Bake for 15 minutes, then remove the fish from the heat and let it cool for 5 minutes
6. In a bowl, combine the coleslaw cabbage and the salsa sauce, toss gently
7. Add the mashed avocado, season with salt and pepper
8. Slice the fish and add to the bowl
9. Bake for 14-15 minutes.
10. Serve hot

Bacon and Zucchini Muffins

Ingredients:

- Salt – 1/2 teaspoon

- Ground turmeric – 1 teaspoon

- Slices of bacon, pastured, diced – 5

- Baking powder – 1 teaspoon

- Apple cider vinegar – 1/2 tablespoon

- Collagen peptides – 1 scoop

- Grated zucchini – 2 cups

- Green onion, chopped – 1

- Thyme sprigs leaves removed – 2

- Coconut flour – 1/2 cup

- Eggs, pastured – 7

Directions:

1. Set oven to 350 degrees F and let preheat until muffins are ready to bake.
2. Take a medium frying pan, place it over medium heat, add bacon pieces, and cook for 3 to 5 minutes until crispy.
3. Then transfer cooked bacon in a large bowl, add remaining ingredients and stir until well combined.
4. Take an eight cups silicon muffin tray, grease the cups with avocado oil and then evenly scoop the prepared batter in them.
5. Place the muffin tray into the oven and bake the muffins for 30 minutes or until thoroughly cooked and the top is nicely golden brown.
6. When done, take out muffins from the tray and cool on the wire rack.

7. Place muffins in a large freezer bag or wrap each muffin with a foil and store them in the refrigerator for four days or in the freezer for up to 3 months.

8. When ready to serve, microwave muffins for 45 seconds to 1 minute or until thoroughly heated.

Blueberry Pancake Bites

Ingredients:

- Swerve Sweetener – 1/4 cup

- Cinnamon – 1/4 teaspoon

- Vanilla extract, unsweetened – 1/2 teaspoon

- Butter, grass-fed, unsalted, melted – 1/4 cup

- Eggs, pastured – 4

- Water – 1/3 cup

- Frozen blueberries – 1/2 cup

- Coconut flour – 1/2 cup

- Baking powder – 1 teaspoon

- Salt – 1/2 teaspoon

Directions:

1. Set oven to 350 degrees F and let preheat until muffins are ready to bake.

2. Crack the eggs in a bowl, add vanilla and sweetener, whisk using an immersion blender until blended and then blend in salt, cinnamon, butter, baking powder, and flour until incorporated and smooth batter comes together.

3. Let the batter sit for 10 minutes or until thickened and then blend in water until combined.

4. Take a 25 cups silicone mini-muffin tray, grease the cups with avocado oil, then evenly scoop the prepared batter in them and top with few blueberries, pressing the berries gently into the batter.

5. Place the muffin tray into the oven and bake the muffins for 25 minutes or until thoroughly cooked and the top is nicely golden brown.

6. When done, take out muffins from the tray and cool them on the wire rack.

7. Place muffins in a large freezer bag or evenly divide them in packets and store them in the refrigerator for four days or in the freezer for up to 3 months.

8. When ready to serve, microwave the muffins for 45 seconds to 1 minute or until thoroughly heated.

Pretzels

Ingredients:

- Eggs, Pastured, beaten – 2

- Mozzarella cheese, full-fat, shredded – 3 cups

- Cream cheese, full-fat, cubed – 2 ounces

- Salt – 1 teaspoon

- Almond flour, blanched – 1 1/2 cups

- Coconut sugar – 1/2 teaspoon

- Baking powder – 1 tablespoon

- Xanthan gum – 1/4 teaspoon

- Dry yeast, active – 2 1/4 teaspoon

- Water, lukewarm – 1/4 cup

Directions:

1. Place yeast in a small bowl, add sugar, pour in water, stir until just mixed and let it sit at a warm place for 10 minutes or until frothy.

2. Then pour the yeast mixture in a food processor, add flour, xanthan gums, eggs, and baking powder and pulse for 1 to 2 minutes or until well combined.

3. Take a heatproof bowl, add cream cheese and mozzarella and microwave for 2 minutes or until melted, stirring every 30 seconds until smooth.

4. Add melted cheese into the processed flour mixture and continue blending until the dough comes together, scraping the mixture from the sides of the blender frequently.

5. Transfer the dough into a bowl and then place it in the refrigerator for 20 minutes or until chilled.

6. Meanwhile, set the oven to 400 degrees F and let preheat.

7. Take out the chilled dough from the refrigerator, then divide the dough into six sections and shape each section into a bowl, using oiled hands.

8. Working on one section at a time, first, roll the section into an 18-inches long log, then take one end, loop it around and down across the bottom and loop the other end, in the same manner, crossing over the first loop to form a pretzel.

9. Prepare remaining pretzels in the same manner and place them on a baking sheet lined with parchment sheet.

10. Sprinkle salt over pretzels, pressing down lightly, then place the baking sheet into the oven and bake pretzels for 10 to 12 minutes until nicely golden.

11. When done, cool the pretzels at room temperature, then keep them in a large plastic bag and store in the refrigerator for up to a week or freeze for up to 3 months.

12. When ready to serve, bake the pretzels at 400 degrees F for 6 to 7 minutes until hot.

Deviled Eggs

Ingredients:

- Smoked paprika – ½ teaspoon

- Dijon mustard – 1 tablespoon

- Mayonnaise, full-fat – ¾ cup

- Water – 1 cup

- Organic eggs – 12

- Salt – ½ teaspoon

- Ground black pepper – ½ teaspoon

Directions:

1. Switch on the instant pot, pour in water, insert steamer rack and place eggs on it.

2. Shut instant pot with its lid, sealed completely, press manual button and cook eggs for 5 minutes on high pressure.

3. When done, let the pressure release naturally for 5 minutes, then do a quick pressure release and open the instant pot.

4. Transfer eggs into a large bowl containing ice-chilled water for 5 minutes, then peel them and cut each egg into half.

5. Transfer egg yolk from each egg into a bowl, add mustard and mayonnaise, season with salt and black pepper and stir until mixed.

6. Spoon the yolk filling into the egg white shells and then sprinkle with paprika.

7. Serve immediately.

Asparagus Fries

Ingredients:

- Chopped parsley – 2 tablespoons

- Parmesan cheese, grated and full-fat – ½ cup

- Organic eggs, beaten – 2

- Mayonnaise, full-fat – 3 tablespoon

- Medium organic asparagus spears – 10

- Organic roasted red pepper, chopped – 1 tablespoon

- Almond flour – ¼ cup

- Garlic powder – ½ teaspoon

- Smoked paprika – ½ teaspoon

Directions:

1. Set oven to 425 degrees F and preheat.
2. Meanwhile, place cheese in a food processor, add garlic and parsley and pulse for 1 minute until fine mixture comes together.
3. Add almond flour, pulse for 30 seconds until just mixed, then tip the mixture into a bowl and season with paprika.
4. Crack eggs into a shallow dish and whisk until beaten.
5. Working on one asparagus spear at a time, first dip into the egg mixture, then coat with parmesan mixture and place it on a baking sheet.
6. Dip and coat more asparagus in the same manner, then arrange them on a baking sheet, 1-inch apart, and bake in the oven for

10 minutes or until asparagus is tender and nicely golden brown.

7. Meanwhile, place mayonnaise in a bowl, add red pepper and whisk until combined and chill the dip into the refrigerator until required.

8. Serve asparagus with prepared dip.

Cucumber Spinach Smoothie

Ingredients:

- MCT oil – 2 tablespoons

- Drops of liquid stevia – 12

- Coconut milk, full-fat and unsweetened – 1 cup

- Ice cubes – 7

- Organic cucumber, peeled and cubed – 2.5 ounces

- Handfuls of organic spinach – 2

- Xanthan gum – ¼ teaspoon

Directions:

1. Place all the ingredients in a food processor or blender and pulse for 1 to 2 minutes or until well combined and smooth.
2. Pour smoothie into a glass and serve immediately.

Blackberry Chocolate Shake

Ingredients:

- Drops of liquid stevia – 12

- Coconut milk, full-fat and unsweetened – 1 cup

- Cubes of ice – 7

- Blackberries, organic – ¼ cup

- Cocoa powder, organic – 2 tablespoons

- Xanthan gum – ¼ teaspoon

- MCT oil – 2 tablespoons

Directions:

1. Place all the ingredients in a food processor or blender and pulse for 1 to 2 minutes or until well combined and smooth.

2. Pour smoothie into a glass and serve immediately.

Bacon-Artichoke Omelet

Ingredients:

- ¼ cup chopped onion

- ½ cup chopped artichoke hearts (canned, packed in water)

- Sea salt

- Freshly ground black pepper

- 6 eggs, beaten

- 2 tablespoons heavy (whipping) cream

- 8 bacon slices, cooked and chopped

- 1 tablespoon olive oil

Directions:

1. Beat together the eggs, heavy cream, and bacon until well blended, and set aside.
2. Take a huge skillet, place it over medium-high heat and add the olive oil.
3. Add the onion and sauté until tender, about 3 minutes.
4. Pour the egg mixture into the skillet, swirling it for 1 minute.
5. Cook the omelet on both sides for 2 minutes.
6. Sprinkle the artichoke hearts on top and flip the omelet. Cook for 4 minutes more until the egg is firm. Flip the omelet over again, so the artichoke hearts are on top.
7. Remove from the heat, cut the omelet into quarters, and season with salt and black pepper. Transfer the omelet to plates and serve.

Jalapeno Hash

Ingredients:

- 6 ounces zucchini, chopped

- 1 teaspoon ground black pepper

- 1 teaspoon butter

- 4 jalapeno peppers, chopped

- ½ cup chicken stock

- 3 ounces bacon, chopped and cooked

Directions:

1. Add jalapeno peppers and zucchini into the Ninja Foodi pot.
2. Put bacon, ground black pepper, butter, and chicken stock.

3. Seal the lid. Set Pressure High. Cook the meat for 5 minutes.

4. Then make natural pressure release for 10 minutes.

5. Once cooked, let the meal chill for a few minutes.

6. Serve with chicken stock and enjoy!

Salad Sandwich

Ingredients:

- 30 g Eden cheese or other cheese (to your taste)

- ½ avocado

- 1 cherry tomato

- 50 g Roman salad

- 15 g butter

Directions:

1. Rinse the lettuce leaves thoroughly and use them as a base for the sandwich.

2. Butter the leaves, chop cheese, avocado, and tomato, and place on the leaves. Place Roman salad over it.
3. Cover with another layer of lettuce leaves. Serve.

Florentine Breakfast Sandwich

Ingredients:

- 1 Versatile Sandwich Round

- 1 tablespoon jarred pesto

- ¼ ripe avocado, mashed

- 1 (¼-inch) thick tomato slice

- 1 (1-ounce) slice fresh mozzarella

- One teaspoon extra-virgin olive oil

- One large egg

- ¼ teaspoon salt

- ¼ teaspoon freshly ground black pepper

Directions:

1. In a small fry pan, heat the olive oil over high heat.

2. When the oil is very hot, crack the egg into the skillet and reduce the heat.

3. Sprinkle the top of the egg with salt and pepper and let it cook for 2 minutes, or until set on bottom.

4. Using a spatula, turn over the egg to cook on the other side to the desired level of doneness (1 to 2 minutes for a runnier yolk, 2 to 3 minutes for a harder yolk).

5. Take away the egg from the pan and keep warm.

6. Cut the sandwich round in half horizontally and toast, if desired.

7. To assemble the sandwich, spread the pesto on a toasted bread half.

8. Top with mashed avocado, the tomato slice, mozzarella, and the cooked egg.

9. Top with the other bread half and eat warm.

Avocado Toast

Ingredients:

- ½ teaspoon garlic powder, sesame seed, caraway seed, or other dried herbs (optional)

- 3 tablespoons extra-virgin olive oil, divided

- 1 medium ripe avocado, peeled, pitted, and sliced

- 2 tablespoons chopped ripe tomato or salsa

- 2 tablespoons ground flaxseed

- ½ teaspoon baking powder

- 2 large eggs

- 1 teaspoon salt, plus more for serving

- ½ teaspoon freshly ground black pepper

Directions:

1. In a small bowl, blend the flaxseed and baking powder, breaking up any lumps in the baking powder. Add the eggs, pepper, salt, and garlic powder (if using) and whisk well.

2. Let it sit for 2 minutes.

3. In a small nonstick skillet, heat one tablespoon olive oil over medium heat. Decant the egg mixture into the skillet and let cook undisturbed until the egg begins to set on the bottom, 2 to 3 minutes.

4. Using a rubber spatula, scrape down the sides to allow uncooked egg to reach the bottom. Cook another 2 to 3 minutes.

5. Once almost set, flip like a pancake and allow the top to cook thoroughly for another 1 to 2 minutes.

6. Remove from the pan and allow to cool slightly.

7. Slice into two pieces.

8. Top each "toast" with avocado slices, additional salt and pepper, chopped tomato, and drizzle with the remaining two tablespoons olive oil.

Caesar Salad Bacon Baskets

Ingredients:

- One/3 cup Ruled.me Caesar dressing

- Salt and pepper to taste

- Two ounces shaved Parmesan cheese

- Eight slices bacon

- 127 grams diced slicing tomato

- 127 grams romaine lettuce

Directions:

1. Oven preheats to 400 ° F. Get the bacon slices halved.

2. Turn a muffin tin upside down to invert pockets.

3. Cross Two slices of bacon over 4 pockets. Wrap two more slices around each of the sides to make 4 cups.
4. Generally speaking, I try to make some extra from the rest of the bacon pack if some don't work out.
5. Bake for another twenty minutes.
6. It is using a fork to gently lift the baskets of bacon off the plate and then place them back on.
7. Place the bacon in the oven and bake until it looks nice and brown.
8. Allow it cool for some fifteen minutes.
9. Cut the lettuce while the bacon is cooking and blend with the tomato and caesar dressing.
10. Divide the salad between baskets of bacon.
11. Top with the Parmesan cheese shavings.

Tomato Asiago Soup

Ingredients:

- One teaspoon oregano

- ¾ cup shredded Asiago cheese

- One teaspoon minced garlic

- Pepper and salt to taste

- One can tomato paste

- One cup heavy whipping cream

- ¼ cup of water

Directions:

1. Place the garlic and tomato paste in a saucepan.

2. Turn the heat on to medium, then pour in the cream.

3. Take the mixture to a boil as you whisk.

4. When it is hot, slowly throw in your Asiago cheese. This will begin to thicken.

5. Bring in the water and cook for 4 to five minutes. Serve with pepper. You may also add some green onions.

6. This makes a total of four servings of Tomato Asiago Soup. Each serving comes out to be

Garlic and Herb Monkey "Bread"

Ingredients:

- One teaspoon garlic powder

- ¼ teaspoon dried basil

- Two tablespoons butter, melted

- One tablespoon chopped fresh basil

- ¾ cup shredded mozzarella cheese

- Two baby eggplants end removed and cubed

Directions:

1. Preheat oven to 375 ° F. Combine the dried basil and garlic powder and add to the butter.

2. At the bottom of each mini bundt pan, layer 7-10 cubes of eggplant.

3. Sprinkle a layer of mozzarella cheese with around One teaspoon of the butter garlic mixture over each layer of eggplant and drizzle.

4. Don't worry about being specific, because all of it will bake together!

5. Follow with another layer of eggplant and cheese and any remaining garlic butter.

6. Cover with the remaining cheese and bake for approximately 20 minutes, or until it is brown.

7. Leave the pans to cool for 5 minutes before removing.

8. Serve with low-carb marinara sauce.

Monterey Mug Melt

Ingredients:

- 1.5 ounces pepper jack cheese, shredded

- 1.5 tablespoons diced green chiles

- Two ounces roast beef deli slices

- One tablespoon sour cream

Directions:

1. Cover one-third of the roasted beef at the bottom of your platter. I like breaking up the roasted beef into smaller pieces.
2. Spread 1⁄2 cubic lb of sour cream carefully.
3. Spread the green chile 1⁄2 tablespoon out.
4. Layer on 1⁄2 ounce of the pepper jack cheese.

5. Repeat with another layer of beef, cheese, chile, and sour cream.

6. Term it off with a roast beef plate, the last 1/2 ounce of cheese, and the last tbsp of green chili.

7. Microwave the cheese for one to two minutes before it melts.

Keto Mug Lasagna

Ingredients:

- 3 ounces whole milk mozzarella

- Two tablespoons whole milk ricotta

- 3 tablespoons Rao's marinara

- 1/3 (65 g) zucchini

Directions:

1. Chop the zucchini into thin sheets of parchment. A very sharp knife, or a mandolin, can be used.
2. Add a teaspoon of the marinara to the bottom of your bowl.
3. Layer on the zucchini.
4. Spread out one tablespoon of ricotta.

5. Add another Tbsp. of Marinara.

6. Place on the second layer of zucchini, another ricotta tablespoon, any remaining zucchini, and then the last marinara spoon.

7. Top mozzarella with.

8. Microwave it for 3 to 4 minutes, depending on your microwave strength. You can sprinkle on a little parmesan cheese or oregano if you like.

KETO BACON WRAPPED CHICKEN
TENDERS WITH RANCH

Ingredients:

- One/Two cup ranch dressing

- Pepper and salt, to taste

- Twenty-4 ounces chicken tenders

- Ten ounces bacon

Directions:

1. Oven preheats to 400 degrees Fahrenheit. Season with salt and pepper on chicken tenders, then wrap bacon around every slice of tenderloin.

2. Put the chicken on a baking sheet and bake for thirty to forty minutes, or until the chicken cooked through.

3. Serve alongside with ranch dressing.

INSTANT POT NO-NOODLE KETO LASAGNA

Ingredients:

- ½ cup Parmesan cheese

- Two large eggs

- One cup of water

- Twenty-five ounces low-carb marinara sauce

- Eight ounces sliced mozzarella

- One pound ground beef

- Two cloves garlic, minced

- One small onion, diced

- 1½ cups ricotta cheese

Directions:

1. Switch on the sauté setting to the Instant Pot. Brown the ground beef, onion, and garlic.
2. The ricotta cheese, parmesan, and eggs are mixed in a separate bowl.
3. Turn off Instant Pot.
4. Take the meat off the Instant Pot and scrape the grease.
5. Mix the marinara in the cooked beef, and save some for the lasagna layer.
6. Use a small springform pan that fits into your Instant Pot, wrapped around the bottom with aluminum foil.
7. Layer the meat, mozzarella, and ricotta. Continue layering until there are no ingredients left.
8. The final layer should be the marinara sauce, which is reserved.

9. Cover the pan loosely with aluminum foil.

10. Pour one cup of water into the Instant Pot. Add the rack then cover it with the springform plate.

11. Close your Instant Pot lid.

12. Close the valve then cook for nine minutes on high pressure.

13. Perform a quick release once done, then serve.

KETO CHEESE SOUFFLÉ

Ingredients:

- Two tablespoons butter
- 1½ tablespoons almond flour
- ¼ teaspoon salt
- Two teaspoons Dijon mustard
- ½ cup shredded cheddar cheese
- 1/3 cup unsweetened almond milk
- 3 tablespoons grated Parmesan cheese
- 3 separated large eggs

Directions:

1. Preheat the oven until 350F. Grease the insides of the ramekins that you'll use.
2. Melt the butter in a saucepan over medium to low heat.

3. Add the almond meal and salt until well mixed. It will densify a little, however, not as much as a higher carb roux.

4. Whisk in the mustard and almond milk, then keep simmering for 5 minutes or until the mixture has thickened a little more.

5. Remove from heat and mix in the cheese of Cheese Parmesan.

6. Whisk in the yolks of the shells, and do not curdle them.

7. Use a mixer to beat the egg whites until stiff peaks develop.

8. Fold gently into a mixture of eggs and cheese.

9. Divide the ramekins into the souffle batter then top with the remaining Parmesan cheese.

10. Then bake the ramekins for 15-20 minutes, or until puffy and crispy. Serve straight away.

APPLE AND SEMOLINA DESSERT

Ingredients:

- 1 cup of sugar

- 6 apples

- 1 cup of semolina

Directions:

1. Peel the apples and grate them.
2. In a bowl for the Oven put in layers, apple, semolina and sugar, successively, and take to soft oven for 20 minutes.

EXOTIC SALAD

Ingredients:

- 3 tablespoons of vinegar

- apples

- 2 tablespoons of honey

- ½ cup evaporated milk

- ¼ cup of oil

- salt and pepper

- 200 g of mixed lettuce

- 200 g of spinach leaves

- 1 tangerine

- 50 g of toasted almonds and cut into sheets (optional)

- 1 sliced avocado

- ALIÑO

Directions:

1. Place the spinach and the vegetables in a salad bowl lettuce chopped by hand, mix, put on it the sliced avocado, the segments of tangerines and almonds.
2. Prepare the dressing mixing all the ingredients in the juicer.
3. Pour over the salad at the moment of serving.

MONGOLIAN MEAT WITH CHAUFAN RICE

Ingredients:

- 1 red pepper and 1 green pepper

- 1 green bell pepper

- ¾ cup of water

- salt, full dressing, pepper

- 250 g of post steak

- 1 onion

- 2 scallions

Directions:

1. Chop the onion in feather, julienne the stems

2. green onions and thinly sliced the part

3. white, in julienne the peppers and in slices the

4. chili. Sauté everything in a deep pan or wook. One

5. Once they are soft, add the water and cover the

6. Frying pan to give juice. On the other hand cut the meat

7. in a triangular shape and grill. Once

8. ready to be seasoned with salt, pepper and full dressing. Join

9. both preparations. Correct the seasoning and add

CHAUFAN RICE

Ingredients:

- fine minced pork or chicken

- salt

- ½ onion

- 2 cups of long grain rice

- 2 eggs

- chives leaves

Directions:

1. Cut the onion into squares and fry.

2. Before to brown add the rice and stir-fry, then add 4 cups of boiling water, salt and cook on fire low.

3. Beat the eggs with a fork, cook them in a Teflon pan, in the shape of a pancake,

4. not to gild.

5. After it cools down, cut into strips in a chopping board.

6. Cooking the meat on the grill and cut. Finely chop the chives leaves. When

7. the rice is ready, gather all the ingredients and mix well.

CELERY SALAD

Ingredients:

- salt, oil and lemon

- 4 cups of celery

Directions:

1. Chop the celery in diagonal rounds, in this way preserves the fiber and does not require unraveling.
2. Dressing.

RISPY CHICKEN WITH MASHED POTATOES

Ingredients:

- ½ liter of chicken broth

- parsley and thyme

- salt and pepper

- 4 whole chicken truffles

- 40 g of breadcrumbs

- 40 g of ground almonds

- 4 tablespoons of chopped herbs

Directions:

1. Clean the chicken, remove the skin and add salt and pepper.
2. Arrange it on a rack in a can of oven. Mix the breadcrumbs, almonds and
3. herbs and cover the chicken with these forming a crust. Place the broth as a cooking base chicken along with the herbs to be flavored.
4. Cook in a preheated and moderate oven, for approximately 40 minutes.

PURÉ DE PAPAS

Ingredients:

- 2 tablespoons of margarine

- 300 ml of skimmed milk

- 6 regular potatoes

- salt

Directions:

1. Peel the potatoes and cook in salted water for 20 minutes, from the time the water boils.

2. Then to go through the mash press, being hot potatoes.

3. Add margarine and blend electric until the potato is soft.

4. Test the salt and add if necessary.

5. Heat the puree in the pot and continue beating with the mixer, add the warm milk slowly.

6. Serve when the puree is boiling.

7. To reheat the mash, you must to be made in a pot, not in a microwave, to be beaten with a spoon wood and add warm milk again from be necessary.

Crunchy Keto Cereal w/ Strawberries

Ingredients:

- Stevia

- Ground Cinnamon

- Parchment Paper or Coconut Oil

- 1 package of Bob's Red Mill Flaked Coconut

- 2 medium sized Strawberries

- Unsweetened Almond Milk

Directions:

1. Preheat your oven to 350 degrees.
2. Line your cookie sheet with your parchment paper. If no parchment paper grease your cooking sheet using coconut oil.

3. Pour your coconut flakes on your cookie sheet.

4. Cook in your oven for approximately 5 minutes.

5. Shuffle flakes around and continue cooking until they are a lightly toasted and lightly tan.

6. Take your flakes out of your oven.

7. Sprinkle them lightly with cinnamon. Can also sprinkle lightly with Stevia.

8. Throw your toasted chips in your bowl and pour your almond milk over them.

9. Slice up 2 strawberries as the garnish on top.

10. Serve!

Berry & Chicken Summer Salad

Ingredients:

- 6 Diced Strawberries

- 3 tablespoons of Raspberry Balsamic Vinegar

- 2 cups of Spinach

- 1/2 cup of Chopped Walnuts

- 3 tablespoons of Crumbled Feta Cheese

- 1 Chicken Breast

- 3/4 cup of Blueberries

Directions:

1. Cut your chicken breast up into small-sized cubes and cook in your pan. When done place on your plate to cool off.
2. Gather your other ingredients and add them to your large-sized bowl. Add your dressing.
3. Add your chicken and toss your salad.
4. Serve!

Grilled Halloumi Salad

Ingredients:

- Handful of Baby Arugula

- Olive Oil

- Balsamic Vinegar

- Salt

- 5 Grape Tomatoes

- 1 Persian Cucumber

- 1/2 ounce of Chopped Walnuts

- 3 ounces of Halloumi Cheese

Directions:

1. Cut your halloumi cheese into approximately 1/3-inch sized slices.

2. Grill your slices for approximately 3 to 5 minutes on both sides.

3. Should have nice grill marks on each side.

4. Prep your salad by washing then cutting your vegetables.

5. Cut your tomatoes in half and cut your cucumbers into smaller slices.

6. Chop your walnuts and add them in your salad bowl.

7. Wash your baby arugula and add to your bowl.

8. Arrange your grilled halloumi cheese on top of your salad.

9. Add some salt.

10. Dress your salad with your balsamic vinegar and olive oil.

11. Serve!

Grilled chicken skewers

Ingredients:

- 1 zucchini, cut into quarters

- salt

- pepper

- 2 teaspoons of Italian herbs

- 1 tbsp sesame oil

- Shish kebab skewers

- 200 g cherry tomatoes

- 1 onion, quartered

- 200 g chicken, diced

- 1 bell pepper, cut into cubes

Directions:

1. Place the skewers in the water for 10 minutes to soak.
2. Mix the oil with the spices and let the meat marinate in it for 10 minutes.
3. Take the skewers out of the water and place the meat with the vegetables alternately on the skewers.
4. Heat the grill and coat the ingredients on the skewers with the marinade.
5. Cook on the grill for 10 minutes. The meat can be pushed with your fingers when it is done.

Golden fish

Ingredients:

- 20 g pine nuts, toasted

- 1 bunch of parsley, chopped

- salt

- pepper

- ½ bunch of dill, chopped

- 2 shallots, chopped

- 1 lemon, organic

- 100 g sour cream

- 300 g Swiss chard

- 2 salmon fillets, a 100 g

Directions:

1. Wash the chard and cut it into strips.

2. Heat a pan and add the Swiss chard and shallots with the spices.

3. Rub the lemon peel and squeeze out the juice.

4. Switch the oven to 180 ° C fan oven.

5. Prepare a baking dish.

6. Pass the contents of the pan through a sieve to drain and collect the brew.

7. Mix the sour cream with lemon juice, lemon zest, herbs and the stock from the pan.

8. Season the salmon fillets and fry them vigorously on both sides.

9. Layer the vegetables with the salmon and pour the cream on top.

10. Scatter the pine nuts on top and cook the casserole in the oven for 15 minutes.

Salmon on a green bed

ingredients:

- 2 tbsp red wine vinegar

- 1 teaspoon mustard

- 2 tbsp sesame oil

- salt

- pepper

- 4 radishes, sliced

- 100 g cocktail tomatoes, halved

- 2 salmon fillets, 100g each

- 200 g lamb's lettuce

Directions:

1. Wash the lettuce and let it drain.

2. Clean the salmon fillets and let them sear on both sides in the pan for 4 minutes.

3. Take the lettuce as well as the radishes and tomatoes and arrange them on a platter, place the salmon in the bed of lettuce.

4. Mix a dressing of oil, vinegar, mustard, salt and pepper and drizzle it over the plate.

Salmon roll

Ingredients:

- 200 g smoked salmon

- 100 g cream cheese, herbs

- 100 g Gouda cheese, grated

- 2 eggs

- 200 g creamed spinach, thawed

Directions:

1. Please preheat your oven to 180 ° C fan oven and prepare a baking sheet with baking paper.

2. Mix the spinach with the eggs.

3. Put this mixture on the baking sheet, spread out and sprinkle with the cheese.

4. Put the tray in the oven for 15 minutes, then let the dough cool down.

5. Loosen the cream cheese and spread it on the dough, place the salmon on top and roll everything up.

6. Let this roll rest in the refrigerator for 4 hours.

7. Cut into slices before serving.

Shrimp pan

Ingredients:

- salt

- 1 clove of garlic, pressed

- 1 tbsp peanut oil

- pepper

- 2 tbsp lemon juice

- 150 g cocktail prawns, ready to cook

- 3 zucchini, cut into pieces

- 3 tomatoes, cut into pieces

- 200 g feta, diced

- 6 olives, chopped

- 1/2 bunch of basil, leaves

Directions:

1. Take a pan and heat the oil in it.
2. Fry the prawns with the garlic and spices.
3. Now fold in the vegetables and let everything simmer for 10 minutes.
4. Fold in the feta, stir everything and turn off the heat.
5. Let everything stand for 3 minutes.
6. Then sprinkle with the basil and serve.

Trout on coconut pillows

Ingredients:

- 1 egg

- 1 cucumber, chopped

- 1 clove of garlic, pressed

- ½ iceberg lettuce, cut into strips

- 2 tbsp lemon juice

- 1 teaspoon vinegar

- salt

- pepper

- 50g coconut flour

- 100 g trout, smoked

- 2 Camembert, nature

Directions:

1. Spread the salad on a serving plate.
2. Mix the yoghurt with the garlic and cucumber as well as salt, pepper, lemon juice and vinegar and drizzle this over the salad.
3. Beat the egg in a deep plate.
4. Dip the camembert first in the egg, then in the coconut flour and press it down firmly.
5. Heat a non-stick pan and fry the camembert until crispy.
6. Place on the salad and divide the trout in between.

Tender Creamy Scallops

Ingredients:

- ½ cup grated parmesan cheese

- 1 cup heavy cream

- 2 tbsp. ghee butter

- Salt and black pepper to taste

- 8 fresh sea scallops

- 4 bacon slices

Directions:

1. Heat the butter in a skillet at medium-high heat

2. Add the bacon and cook for 4-5 minutes each side (till crispy)

3. Moved to a paper towel to remove the excess fat

4. Lower the heat to medium, sprinkle with more butter. Put the heavy cream and parmesan cheese, season with salt and pepper

5. Reduce the heat to low and cook for 8-10 minutes, constantly stirring, until the sauce thickens

6. In another skillet, heat the ghee butter over medium-high heat

7. Add the scallops to the skillet, season with salt and pepper. Cook for 2 minutes per side until golden

8. Transfer the scallops to a paper towel

9. Top with the sauce and crumbled bacon

Salmon Cakes

Ingredients:

- 3 tbsp. keto mayo

- 1 tbsp. ghee butter

- 1 tbsp. Dijon mustard

- Salt and ground black pepper to taste

- 6 oz. canned salmon

- 1 large egg

- 2 tbsp. pork rinds

Directions:

1. In a bowl, combine the salmon (drained), pork rinds, egg, and half of the mayo, season with salt and pepper. Mix well
2. With the salmon mixture, form the cakes
3. Heat the ghee butter in a skillet over medium-high heat
4. Place the salmon cakes in the skillet and cook for about 3 minutes per side.
5. Moved to a paper towel to get rid of excess fat
6. In a small bowl, combine the remaining half of mayo and the Dijon mustard, mix well
7. Serve the salmon cakes with the mayo-mustard sauce

Salmon with Mustard Cream

Ingredients:

- 2 tbsp. fresh cilantro, minced

- 2 tbsp. ghee butter

- ½ tsp garlic powder

- Salt and pepper to taste

- 2 salmon fillets

- ¼ cup keto mayo

- 1 tbsp. Dijon mustard

Directions:

1. Preheat the oven to 450F. Grease a baking dish with the ghee butter

2. Season the salmon with salt and pepper and put in the baking dish

3. In a mixing bowl, put and combine the Dijon mustard, mayo, parsley, and garlic powder. Stir well

4. Top the salmon fillets with the mustard sauce

5. Bake for 10 minutes

Easy Chicken Tacos

Ingredients:

- 1 clove garlic, minced

- 1 cup tomato puree

- 1/2 cup salsa

- 2 slices bacon, chopped

- 1 pound ground chicken

- 1 ½ cups Mexican cheese blend

- 1 tablespoon Mexican seasoning blend

- 2 teaspoons butter, room temperature

- 2 small-sized shallots, peeled and finely
  chopped

Directions:

1. In a saucepan, put butter then melt in over a moderately high flame.

2. Now, cook the shallots until tender and fragrant.

3. Then, sauté the garlic, chicken, and bacon for about 5 minutes, stirring continuously and crumbling with a fork.

4. Add the in Mexican seasoning blend.

5. Fold in the tomato puree and salsa; continue to simmer for 5 to 7 minutes over medium-low heat; reserve.

6. Line a baking pan with wax paper. Place 4 piles of the shredded cheese on the baking pan and gently press them down with a wide spatula to make "taco shells."

7. Bake in the preheated oven at 365 degrees F for 6 to 7 minutes or until melted.

8. Allow these taco shells to cool for about 10 minutes.

Cheesy Bacon-Wrapped Chicken with Asparagus Spears

Ingredients:

- From the cupboard

- 4 tablespoons olive oil, divided

- Salt, to taste

- Freshly ground black pepper, to taste

- 4 chicken breasts

- 8 bacon slices

- 1 pound (454 g) asparagus spears

- 2 tablespoons fresh lemon juice

- ½ cup Manchego cheese, grated

Directions:

1. Set the oven to 400ºF. Line a baking sheet using parchment paper, then grease with 1 tablespoon olive oil.
2. Put the chicken breasts in a large bowl, and sprinkle with salt and black pepper.
3. Toss to combine well.
4. Wrap every chicken breast with 2 slices of bacon.
5. Place the chicken on the baking sheet, then bake in the preheated oven for 25 minutes or until the bacon is crispy.
6. Preheat the grill to high, then brush with the remaining olive oil.
7. Place the asparagus spears on the grill grate, and sprinkle with salt.
8. Grill for 5 minutes or until fork-tender.

9. Flip the asparagus frequently during the grilling.

10. Transfer the bacon-wrapped chicken breasts to four plates, drizzle with lemon juice, and scatter with Manchego cheese.

11. Spread the hot asparagus spears on top to serve.

Bacon-Wrapped Chicken with Cheddar Cheese

Ingredients:

- 4 garlic cloves, crushed

- ½ cup Cheddar cheese, grated

- 2 large chicken breasts, each cut into 6 pieces

- 6 slices of streaky bacon, each cut in half widthways

From the cupboard:

- Freshly ground black pepper, to taste

- 1 tablespoon olive oil

- Salt, to taste

Directions:

1. Grease the insert of the slow cooker with olive oil.
2. Wrap each piece of chicken breast with each half of the bacon slice, and arrange them in the slow cooker.
3. Sprinkle with garlic, salt, and black pepper.
4. Put the lid and then cook on LOW for 4 hours.
5. Set the oven to 350ºF (180ºC).
6. Transfer the cooked bacon-wrapped chicken to a baking dish, then scatter with cheese.
7. Cook in the preheated oven for 5 minutes or until the cheese melts.
8. Take it off from the oven and serve warm.

Capocollo and Garlic Chicken

Ingredients:

- Coarse sea salt, to taste

- Ground black pepper, to taste

- 1/2 teaspoon smoked paprika

- 2 pounds chicken drumsticks, skinless and boneless, butterflied

- 10 thin slices of capocollo

- 1 garlic clove, peeled and halved

Directions:

1. Rub garlic halves over the surface of chicken drumsticks.

2. Season with paprika, salt, and black pepper.

129

3. Place a slice of capocollo on each chicken drumsticks and roll them up; secure with kitchen twine.

4. Bake in the oven at 410°F for 30 to 35 minutes until your chicken begins to brown.

5. Bon appétit!

Super Herbed Fish

Ingredients:

- 1 thyme sprig

- 1 teaspoon Dijon mustard

- ¼ teaspoon garlic powder

- Pinch of salt

- Pinch of pepper

- 1 ½ cups water

- 1 tablespoon chopped basil

- 2 teaspoons lime zest

- 1 tablespoon lime juice

- 1 tablespoon olive oil

- 1 4-ounce fish fillet

- 1 rosemary sprig

Directions:

1. Season the fish with salt and paper. Arrange on a piece of parchment paper and sprinkle with zest.
2. Whisk together the oil, juice, and mustard in a mixing bowl and brush over.
3. Top with the herbs.
4. Wrap the fish with the parchment paper.
5. Wrap the wrapped fish in an aluminum foil.
6. Arrange Instant Pot over a dry platform in your kitchen.
7. Open its top lid and switch it on.
8. In the pot, pour water.
9. Arrange a trivet or steamer basket inside that came with Instant Pot.

10. Now place/arrange the foil over the trivet/basket.
11. Close the lid to create a locked chamber; make sure that safety valve is in locking position.
12. Find and press "MANUAL" cooking function; timer to 5 minutes with default "HIGH" pressure mode.
13. Allow the pressure to build to cook the ingredients.
14. After cooking time is over press "CANCEL" setting.
15. Find and press "QPR" cooking function. This setting is for quick release of inside pressure.
16. Slowly open the lid, take out the cooked recipe in serving plates or serving bowls, and enjoy the keto recipe.

Turkey Avocado Chili

Ingredients:

- 1 (4-ounce) can green chilies with liquid

- 2 tablespoons Worcestershire sauce

- 1 tablespoon dried oregano

- ¼ cup red chili powder

- 2 tablespoons (finely ground) cumin

- Salt and freshly (finely ground) black pepper, as per taste preference

- 1 pitted and sliced avocado, peeled

- 2 ½ pounds lean (finely ground) turkey

- 2 cups diced tomatoes

- 2-ounce tomato paste, sugar-free

- 1 tablespoon olive oil

- ½ chopped large yellow onion

- 8 minced garlic cloves

Directions:

1. Arrange Instant Pot over a dry platform in your kitchen.
2. Open its top lid and switch it on.
3. Find and press cooking function; add the oil in it and allow it to heat.
4. In the pot, add the onions; cook (while stirring) until turns translucent and softened for around 4-5 minutes.
5. Add the garlic and cook for about 1 minute.

6. Add the turkey and cook for about 8-9 minutes. Stir in remaining ingredients except for the avocado.

7. Close the lid to create a locked chamber; make sure that safety valve is in locking position.

8. Find and press "MEAT/STEW" cooking function; timer to 35 minutes with default "HIGH" pressure mode.

9. Allow the pressure to build to cook the ingredients.

10. After cooking time is over press "CANCEL" setting. Find and press "NPR" cooking function. This setting is for the natural release of inside pressure, and it takes around 10 minutes to release pressure slowly.

11. Slowly open the lid, take out the cooked recipe in serving plates or serving bowls, top

with the avocado slices, and enjoy the keto recipe.

Cheesy Tomato Shrimp

Ingredients:

- 1 jalapeno, diced

- 1 onion, diced

- 1 cup shredded cheddar cheese

- 1 teaspoon minced garlic

- 2 tablespoons olive oil

- ½ cup veggie broth

- ¼ cup chopped cilantro

- 2 tablespoons lime juice

- 1 ½ pounds shrimp, peeled and deveined

- 1 ½ pounds tomatoes, chopped

Directions:

1. Arrange Instant Pot over a dry platform in your kitchen.
2. Open its top lid and switch it on.
3. Find and press "SAUTE" cooking function; add the oil in it and allow it to heat.
4. In the pot, add the onions; cook (while stirring) until turns translucent and softened for around 2-3 minutes.
5. Add garlic and sauté for 30-60 seconds.
6. Stir in the broth, cilantro, and tomatoes.
7. Close the lid to create a locked chamber; make sure that safety valve is in locking position.

8. Find and press "MANUAL" cooking function; timer to 9 minutes with default "HIGH" pressure mode.

9. Allow the pressure to build to cook the ingredients.

10. After cooking time is over press "CANCEL" setting.

11. Find and press "NPR" cooking function.

12. This setting is for the natural release of inside pressure, and it takes around 10 minutes to release pressure slowly.

13. Add the shrimps.

14. Close the top lid to create a locked chamber; make sure that safety valve is in locking position.

15. Find and press "MANUAL" cooking function; timer to 2 minutes with default "HIGH" pressure mode.

16. Allow the pressure to build to cook the ingredients.

17. After cooking time is over press "CANCEL" setting.

18. Find and press "NPR" cooking function.

19. This setting is for the natural release of inside pressure, and it takes around 10 minutes to release pressure slowly.

20. Slowly open the lid, take out the cooked recipe in serving plates or serving bowls, top with the cheddar, and enjoy the keto recipe.

Cajun Rosemary Chicken

Ingredients:

- 2 rosemary sprigs

- 1 tablespoon coconut oil

- 1/4 teaspoon pepper

- 1 1/2 cups chicken broth

- 2 teaspoons Cajun seasoning

- 1 lemon, halved

- 1 yellow onion, make quarters

- 1 teaspoon garlic salt

- 1 medium chicken

Directions:

1. Season the chicken with garlic salt, pepper, and Cajun seasoning.
2. Stuff the lemon, onion, and rosemary in the chicken's cavity.
3. Arrange Instant Pot over a dry platform in your kitchen.
4. Open its top lid and switch it on.
5. Find and press "SAUTE" cooking function; add the oil in it and allow it to heat.
6. In the pot, add the meat; cook (while stirring) until turns evenly brown from all sides.
7. Add the broth; gently stir to mix well.
8. Close the lid to create a locked chamber; make sure that safety valve is in locking position.

9. Find and press "MANUAL" cooking function; timer to 25 minutes with default "HIGH" pressure mode.

10. Allow the pressure to build to cook the ingredients.

11. After cooking time is over press "CANCEL" setting.

12. Find and press "NPR" cooking function.

13. This setting is for the natural release of inside pressure, and it takes around 10 minutes to release pressure slowly.

14. Slowly open the lid, take out the cooked recipe in serving plates or serving bowls, and enjoy the keto recipe.

Kale Chips

Ingredients:

- Olive oil – 2 tablespoons

- Large bunch of organic kale – 1

- Seasoned salt – 1 tablespoon

Directions:

1. Set oven to 350 degrees F and preheat.

2. Meanwhile, separate kale leaves from its stem, rinse the leaves under running water, then drain completely by using a vegetable spinner.

3. Wipe kale leaves with paper towels to remove excess water, then transfer them into a large plastic bag and add oil.

4. Seal the plastic bag, turn it upside down until kale is coated with oil and then spread kale leaves on a large baking sheet.

5. Place the baking sheet into the oven and bake for 12 minutes or until its edges are nicely golden brown.

6. Remove baking sheet from the oven, season kale with salt and serve.

Roasted Nuts

Ingredients:

- Red chili powder – 1 teaspoon

- Ground cumin – 1 teaspoon

- Coconut oil – 1 tablespoon

- Pecans – 8 ounce

- Salt – 1 teaspoon

Directions:

1. Place a frying pan over medium heat, add all the ingredients and stir until mixed.
2. Cook pecans for 5 minutes or until warm through and then remove the pan from heat.
3. Serve straight away.

Guacamole

Ingredients:

- Tomato salsa, organic – 2 tablespoons

- Lime juice, organic – 1 tablespoon

- Bunch of organic cilantro – ½

- Organic avocados, pitted – 2

- Medium organic red onion, peeled and sliced – 1/3

- Medium organic jalapeño, deseeded and diced – 1

- Salt – ½ teaspoon

- Ground pepper – ½ teaspoon

Directions:

1. Cut each avocado into half, remove its pit and slice its flesh horizontally and vertically.
2. Scoop out the flesh of the avocado, place it in a bowl and add onion, jalapeno, and lime juice then stir until well mixed.
3. Season with salt and black pepper, add salsa and stir with a fork until avocado is mash to desired consistency.
4. Fold in cilantro and serve.

Chocolate Avocado Ice Cream

Ingredients:

- Coconut milk, full-fat and unsweetened – 1 cup

- Heavy whipping cream, full-fat – ½ cup

- Squares of chocolate, unsweetened and chopped – 6

- Large organic avocados, pitted – 2

- Erythritol, powdered – ½ cup

- Cocoa powder, organic and unsweetened – ½ cup

- Drops of liquid stevia – 25

- Vanilla extract, unsweetened – 2 teaspoons

Directions:

1. Scoop out the flesh from each avocado, place it in a bowl and add vanilla, milk, and cream and blend using an immersion blender until smooth and creamy.

2. Add remaining ingredients except for chocolate and mix until well combined and smooth.

3. Fold in chopped chocolate and let the mixture chill in the refrigerator for 8 to 12 hours or until cooled.

4. When ready to serve, let ice cream stand for 30 minutes at room temperature, then process it using an ice cream machine as per manufacturer instruction.

5. Serve immediately.

Lemon–Olive Oil Breakfast Cakes with Berry Syrup

Ingredients:

For the Pancakes

- 6 tablespoon extra-virgin olive oil, divided

- 2 large eggs

- Zest and juice of 1 lemon

- ½ teaspoon almond or vanilla extract

- 1 cup almond flour

- 1 teaspoon baking powder

- ¼ teaspoon salt

For the Berry Sauce

- ½ teaspoon vanilla extract

- 1 cup of frozen mixed berries

- 1 tablespoon water or lemon juice, plus more
  if needed

Directions:

1. To Make the Pancakes
2. In a large bowl, blend the almond flour,
   baking powder, salt, and whisk to break any
   clumps.
3. Add the 4 tablespoons olive oil, eggs, lemon
   zest and juice, and almond extract and whisk
   to combine well.
4. In a large skillet, heat 1 tablespoon of olive oil
   and spoon about 2 tablespoons of batter for

each of 4 pancakes. Cook until bubbles begin
to form, 4 to 5 minutes, and flip.

5. Cook another 2 to 3 minutes on the second
    side.
6. Repeat with the remaining 1 tablespoon olive
    oil and batter.
7. To Make the Berry Sauce
8. In a small saucepan, heat the frozen berries,
    water, and vanilla extract over medium-high
    heat for 3 to 4 minutes, until bubbly.
9. Add more water if the mixture is too thick.
    Through the back of a spoon, mash the
    berries and whisk until smooth.

Greek Yogurt Parfait

Ingredients:

- ½ teaspoon vanilla or almond extract (optional)

- ¼ teaspoon ground cinnamon (optional)

- 1 tablespoon ground flaxseed

- 2 tablespoons chopped nuts (walnuts or pecans)

- ½ cup plain whole-milk Greek yogurt

- 2 tablespoons heavy whipping cream

- ¼ cup frozen berries, thawed with juices

Directions:

1. In a small bowl or glass, blend the yogurt, heavy whipping cream, thawed berries in their juice, vanilla or almond extract (if using), cinnamon (if using), flaxseed, and stir well until smooth.
2. Top with chopped nuts and enjoy.

Nut Medley Granola

Ingredients:

- ½ cup melted coconut oil

- 10 drops liquid stevia

- 1 teaspoon ground cinnamon

- ½ teaspoon ground nutmeg

- 2 cups shredded unsweetened coconut

- 1 cup sliced almonds

- 1 cup raw sunflower seeds

- ½ cup raw pumpkin seeds

- ½ cup walnuts

Directions:

1. Preheat the oven to 250°F. Line 2 baking sheets with parchment paper. Set aside.
2. Put together the shredded coconut, almonds, sunflower seeds, pumpkin seeds, and walnuts in a large bowl until mixed.
3. Blend the coconut oil, stevia, cinnamon, and nutmeg until blended.
4. Combine the coconut oil mixture and nut mixture. Utilize your hands to mix until the nuts are well coated.
5. Place the granola mixture on the baking sheets and spread it out evenly.
6. Bake the granola, stir every 10 minutes, until the mixture is golden brown and crunchy, about 1 hour.

7. Move the granola mixture to a large bowl and let it cool, tossing it frequently to break up the large pieces.

8. The granola can be stored in an airtight container in the refrigerator or freezer for up to 1 month.

Frittata

Ingredients:

- 1 cup fresh spinach, arugula, kale, or other leafy greens

- 4 ounces quartered artichoke hearts, rinsed, drained, and thoroughly dried

- 8 cherry tomatoes halved

- ½ cup crumbled soft goat cheese

- 4 large eggs

- 2 tablespoons fresh chopped herbs, such as rosemary, thyme, oregano, basil, or 1 teaspoon dried herbs

- ¼ teaspoon salt

- Freshly ground black pepper

- 4 tablespoons extra-virgin olive oil, divided

Directions:

1. Preheat the oven to broil on low.
2. In a small bowl, blend the eggs, herbs, salt, and pepper and whisk well with a fork. Set aside.
3. In a 4- to 5-inch oven-safe skillet or omelet pan, heat 2 tablespoons of olive oil over medium heat. Add the spinach, artichoke hearts, cherry tomatoes, and sauté until just wilted 1 to 2 minutes.
4. Pour in the egg mixture, then cook undisturbed over medium heat for 3 to 4 minutes, until the eggs begin to set on the bottom.

5. Sprinkle the goat cheese across the top of the egg mixture and transfer the skillet to the oven.

6. Broil for 4 to 5 minutes, or until the frittata is firm in the center and golden brown on top.

7. Remove from the oven and run a rubber spatula around the edge to loosen the sides. Invert onto a large plate or cutting board and slice in half.

8. Serve warm and drizzled with the remaining two tablespoons of olive oil.

Mushroom Frittata

Ingredients:

- 10 large eggs, beaten

- ½ cup crumbled goat cheese

- Sea salt

- Freshly ground black pepper

- 2 tablespoons olive oil

- 1 cup sliced fresh mushrooms

- 1 cup shredded spinach

- 6 bacon slices, cooked and chopped

Directions:

1. Preheat the oven to 350°F.

2. Put an ovenproof skillet and add the olive oil.

3. Fry the mushrooms until they turn lightly brown, about 3 minutes.

4. Add the bacon and spinach then sauté until the greens are wilted about a minute.

5. Add the eggs and cook, lifting the edges of the frittata with a spatula so uncooked egg flows underneath, for 3 to 4 minutes.

6. Season lightly with salt and pepper.

7. Bake until lightly browned, about 15 minutes.

8. Take away the frittata from the oven, and let it stand for 5 minutes.

9. Cut into 6 wedges and serve immediately.

Breakfast Bake

Ingredients:

- 1 tablespoon chopped fresh oregano

- Sea salt

- Freshly ground black pepper

- ½ cup shredded Cheddar cheese

- 1 tablespoon olive oil

- 1-pound preservative-free or homemade sausage

- 8 large eggs

- 2 cups cooked spaghetti squash

Directions:

1. Preheat the oven to 375°F. Put olive oil into a 9-by-13-inch casserole dish and set aside.

2. Place a huge ovenproof skillet over medium-high heat and add the olive oil.

3. Brown the sausage until cooked through, about 5 minutes. While the sausage is cooking, whisk together the eggs, squash, and oregano in a medium bowl. Put a little salt and pepper and set aside.

4. Add the cooked sausage to the egg mixture, stir until just combined, and pour the mixture into the casserole dish.

5. Add a layer of cheese at the top and cover the casserole loosely with aluminum foil.

6. Bake the casserole for 30 minutes, and then take away the foil and bake for another 15 minutes.

7. Allow it to cool for 15 minutes before serving.

KETO GROUND BEEF STROGANOFF

Ingredients:

- Two tablespoon water

- 1¼ cup sour cream

- ½ teaspoon paprika

- One pound 80% lean ground beef

- One tablespoon fresh lemon juice

- Two tablespoon butter

- One clove minced garlic

- Pepper and salt, to taste

- Ten ounces sliced mushrooms

- One tablespoon fresh chopped parsley

Directions:

1. At medium heat, preheat a large skillet, then add the butter.
2. Add the minced garlic when the butter has melted and avoided foaming.
3. Cook the garlic over frequent stirring until it is fragrant, then add the ground beef—season with pepper and salt.
4. Continue to cook the ground beef with a wooden spoon and break up the grounds.
5. Transfer the cooked beef to a saucepan and set aside.
6. Drain much of the fat from the skillet, letting the mushrooms cook just enough on the rim.
7. Switch up the heat to low.
8. Add the chestnuts and water to the saucepan. Continue to cook until the water has halved, and the mushrooms are tender.

9. Put away the mushrooms.

10. Reduce the heat, and then whisk the sour cream and paprika in the skillet.

11. Add the mushrooms and cooked beef back into the saucepan and stir.

12. Then serve in the lemon juice and the parsley.

KETO TEX-MEX OPEN-FACED BURGER

Ingredients:

- Two ounces lettuce

- Two tablespoons pickled jalapeños

- 1/3 cup sour cream

- Pepper and salt, to taste

- One tablespoon taco seasoning

- 2/3 pound ground beef

- 4 tablespoons olive oil

- One-ounce sliced pepper jack cheese

- One large avocado

Directions:

1. Seasoning of ground beef, and taco.

2. Forme a burger patty, season with salt and pepper, then set aside for each serving.

3. Preheat a skillet over medium heat, then cut the olive oil in half.

4. Give the burger patties a few seconds to heat up then add. Cook on either side before they cook the burgers all the way cooked.

5. One burger patty with the pepper jack cheese, avocado, lettuce, jalapenos, and sour cream for each serving plate.

6. Sprinkle the remaining olive oil on top and serve.

7. This makes a total of two servings of Keto Tex-Mex Open-Faced Burger.

8. Each serving comes out to be 749.45 Calories, 5.8g Net Carbs, 66.3g Fats, and 27g Protein.

BACON WRAPPED CHICKEN CORDON BLEU

Ingredients*:*

- Twelve to Fifteen toothpicks

- 4 slices black forest ham

- Eight slices bacon

- Two large boneless skinless chicken breasts

- Two ounces bleu cheese

Directions:

1. Start by trimming the breast meat. I split the two halves and strip extra meat off.

2. Slice any portion of the breast carefully in half lengthwise

3. Place it open when you are done cutting it in half after you get it going. Pay attention to keeping both halves intact. You don't want to cut through all the way, just enough to lay it flat open.

4. Have all the ingredients you want packed. You needn't think about cross-contamination this way.

5. Place a piece of ham on the breast of the chicken and put the cheese in the middle.

6. Turn 1/3 slice of ham over the cheese and fold the remaining 1/3 over to cover

7. Fold the chicken carefully in two, covered with bacon. Take a piece of bacon and stretch it gently through pulling on both ends. Starting at one end, start wrapping in chicken.

8. When you've wrapped the chicken around, take the second piece of bacon and tie it to the top. Secure with toothpicks.

9. Place wrapped chicken in an oven-proof skillet (I prefer using cast iron) filled with butter, coconut oil, or bacon fat.

10. Preheat oven to 325 degrees. Brown bacon on all 4 sides, in a skillet over medium heat.

11. Take the saucepan from the top of the stove and put it in the oven. Cook until chicken is cooked, or for forty-five minutes. Let sit for two minutes, then serve.

Cheddar Bacon Explosion

Ingredients:

- Two teaspoons Mrs. Dash Table Seasoning

- Two ½ cups shredded cheddar cheese

- Thirty slices of bacon

- Five cups raw spinach

- Two tablespoons Tones Southwest Chipotle Seasoning

Directions:

1. Preheat your oven to 375F convection bake.
2. Weave the bacon. Fifteen pieces that are vertical, twelve pieces horizontal, and the extra 3 cut in half, to fill in rest, horizontally.

3. Season your favorite seasoning mix to the bacon.

4. Place the cheese in the bacon, leaving a distance of about One One/Two-inch between the sides.

5. Add your spinach and tap it to compress some. It will help when you roll it up.

6. Slowly roll up your weave, make sure it stays tight and doesn't fall too much through.

7. You might have some cheese falling out, but don't worry.

8. Attach your outdoor seasoning here, if you wish.

9. Foil and apply plenty of salt to a baking dish. This will help catch excess bacon grease, and not allow your oven to smoke.

10. Place your bacon on top of a cooling rack and place it over your baking sheet.

11. Bake for 6ty to seventy minutes, without opening the oven door.

12. Once finished, your bacon should be very crisp to the top.

13. Let cool off for ten to fifteen minutes before attempting to take it out.

14. Slice in pieces, then serve!

Chicken Pesto Roulade

Ingredients:

- 150g Halloumi Cheese

- One tsp. Salt

- One tsp. Pepper

- Two Tbsp. Olive Oil (For Frying)

- 4 Chicken Breasts

- 1/4 cup Pesto

- One Tbsp. Olive Oil

- One Lemon's Zest

- One tsp. Garlic

Directions:

1. Press any extra moisture on your chicken breasts dry. The chicken breasts are pounded into 1/8 "bits.

2. Mix 1/4 cup Pesto along with One Tbsp. Olive Oil. Spread the mixture over the chicken breasts.

3. For each chicken, add salt, pepper, and lemon zest.

4. Fill each chicken breast with sliced Halloumi cheese.

5. I am using butcher string or toothpicks to roll the chicken breasts up and tie them.

6. Oven preheats to 450F.

7. Heat two Tbsp. Olive oil to high heat in cast iron.

8. Sear off either side of the chicken to make sure it gets nice and brown.

9. Bake for 6 to seven minutes until juice runs free.

Keto Kale & Sausage Soup

Ingredients:

- 4 cups of Low-Sodium Chicken Broth

- 3 cups of Chopped Kale

- 1/2 Medium Head Cauliflower (Cut Into Small Florets)

- 1 teaspoon of Sea Salt

- 1/2 teaspoon of Freshly Ground Black Pepper

- 1 pound of Sweet Italian Sausage (Ground)

- 1 Medium Carrot (Peeled & Diced)

- 1 Medium Yellow Onion (Chopped)

- 1 tablespoon of Butter

- 2 cloves of Crushed Garlic

- 1 teaspoon of Dried Oregano

- 2 tablespoons of Red Wine Vinegar

- 1 teaspoon of Dried Rubbed Sage

- 1 teaspoon of Dried Basil

- 1/2 teaspoon of Crushed Red Pepper Flakes

- 1 cup of Heavy Whipping Cream

Directions:

1. Heat your large-sized saucepan or Dutch oven over a medium-high heat.
2. Add your ground sausage, breaking up your meat.
3. Cook, stirring occasionally until browned and cooked through, Should take approximately 5 minutes.

4. Using your slotted spoon, remove your cooked sausage and allow to drain on a plate covered with your paper towels.

5. Discard the drippings, but do not wash your pan.

6. Melt your butter over a medium heat.

7. When the bubbling subsides, add your onion and carrot.

8. Cook until your onion begins to brown on the edges and becomes somewhat translucent.

9. Stir your garlic into your onion and carrot mixture.

10. Cook for approximately 1 minute. Add your red wine vinegar and cook until syrupy, scraping up any browned bits. Should take about 1 minute.

11. Stir in your oregano, basil, sage and red pepper flakes.

12. Pour in your stock and heavy cream. Increase the heat to a medium high.

13. When your soup reaches a simmer, add your cauliflower and turn the heat down to a medium-low.

14. Simmer uncovered until your cauliflower is fork-tender.

15. Should take about 10 minutes.

16. Stir in your kale and cooked sausage.

17. Cook 1 to 2 minutes longer, or until your kale wilts and your sausage is reheated.

18. Season with your salt and pepper.

19. The amount of salt needed may vary due to variation in brands of broth.

20. Serve!

Broccoli Chicken Zucchini Boats

Ingredients:

- 2 tablespoons of Butter

- 1 stalk of Green Onion

- 1 cup of Broccoli

- Salt

- Pepper

- 6 ounces of Shredded Rotisserie Chicken

- 3 ounces of Shredded Cheddar Cheese

- 2 Large Zucchini (Hollowed Out)

- 2 tablespoons of Sour Cream

Directions:

1. Preheat your oven to 400 degrees and cut your zucchini in half lengthwise.

2. The longer the zucchini the better for this specific recipe.

3. Using your spoon, scoop out most of the zucchini until you're left with a shell about 1 centimeter thick.

4. Pour 1 tablespoon of melted butter into each zucchini boat.

5. Season with your salt and pepper and place them in your oven.

6. This allows your zucchini to cook down while you prepare the filling.

7. This should take approximately 20 minutes.

8. Shred your rotisserie chicken using two forks to pull your meat apart.

9. Measure out 6 ounces and save the rest for another meal.

10. Cut up your broccoli florets until they're bite sized.

11. Combine your chicken and broccoli with your sour cream to keep them moist and creamy. Season in this step as well.

12. Once your zucchini has had a chance to cook, take them out and add your chicken and broccoli filling.

13. Sprinkle your cheddar cheese over the top of your chicken and broccoli and pop them back into your oven for an additional 10 to 15 minutes or until your cheese is melted and browning.

14. Garnish with your chopped green onion and enjoy with sour cream or mayo if so desired.

15. Serve!

CPSIA information can be obtained
at www.ICGtesting.com
Printed in the USA
LVHW010510050422
715274LV00011B/491

9 781990 053276